My Diary

A Postpartum Journey from Pain to Purpose

Jane I. Honikman, M.S.

Disclaimer: The information contained in this publication is advisory only and is not intended to replace sound clinical judgment or individualized patient care. The author disclaims all warranties, whether expressed or implied, including any warranty as the quality, accuracy, safety, or suitability of this information for any particular purpose.

ISBN 978-1542616591

Printed in the United States of America

Cover design and book layout: Dowitcher Designs

To obtain copies of this book, please visit:
www.janehonikman.com.

Dedicated to the families, including my own, touched by secrets, lack of social support, and silence surrounding our parenting experiences.

Prologue

It is embarrassing to read what I scribbled into a green Girl Scout autograph book I converted into my first diary as a 12 year old 7th grader. From my first entry in 1958, it is evident that I liked boys. I ranked them; first through third. My thickly penciled handwriting is atrocious. My primary words of prepubescent emotion were "he looked at me" and "I like him." By 9th grade I was writing with a pen into a pink diary with a lock and key. I wrote about my relationships with girls as well as school work and important events such as getting my period, having my braces removed, sleepovers, school dances and, of course, boys. I documented arguments between best friends, our jealousies and long phone calls to resolve our differences. Upon reflection on those days of innocence, it is obvious why I decided to write my postpartum story as a diary.

It is now fifty years since I met the man who fathered our three children. In 1965, he arrived in Palo Alto, California to attend graduate school at Stanford University. It was the summer between my sophomore and junior years at college. We fell in love "on the street where we lived." My Diary entries describe our journey. I did not actually keep a journal over those years. My accumulation of scrapbooks, photo albums and emotional intelligence guided me when I felt ready to write.

My purpose in sharing our story is egocentric. I needed to heal my soul. It reflects my progression from a painful past to purposeful future. My actions were derived from a practical application of lessons learned from experience. I don't believe this is especially unique. Everyone has a story to tell, it is healthy to do so, and it also helps others who can identify with what has been written. I self-published *My Diary* in 2000 in my first book called *Step by Step*. The feedback I received was validating and touching. I had made a difference in the lives of other people. The Diary was removed when that book was updated and published as *Community Support for New Families* in 2013. Now it is time to take the Diary off the shelf, dust it off, and share.

I'll be turning seventy this year. Being open and honest is a good way to celebrate life. Given my genetic history I should have a couple more decades to continue to embrace each day. Thank you, mom and dad. I wouldn't be here without you!

August 1965 ♥

Dear Diary,

I have a secret and I feel so alone. I think I might be pregnant, but I can't believe this could be happening to me. I told my boyfriend I thought I was but he said I couldn't be so I guess maybe I'm not. I'm confused and afraid to tell anyone else. What would they think of me? I'm getting ready to leave for Europe and that part of my life is exhilarating. That's all I'm going to think about and I'll be fine.

September 1965

··

Dear Diary,

I've decided to "talk" to you, dear Diary, while I travel and live overseas. I feel very alone even in the midst of many. It was exciting visiting relatives before meeting up with my college friends in New Year City. Sometimes I imagine myself asking for advice from others but I don't have the courage. The words are stuck deep inside my throat. I can't be pregnant, I don't feel different.

October 1965 🖤

Dear Diary,

Sorry, I haven't been writing, but I haven't wanted to share my sad, scared and secret side even with you. I turned 20 when we were in Amsterdam on our student tour. We arrived in Copenhagen and met our families, mine is wonderful! I'm so used to smiling and pretending that nothing is worrying me that it actually works most of the time. But then I hear that nagging, haunting menace in the back of my mind. I finally saw a doctor and yes, I'm pregnant. I'm a liar and a fool. I hate myself for being so stupid. I've been terrified about hurting everyone I love by telling the truth. I have this secret and I don't want to share it. I keep thinking it will just go away like having a nightmare and then waking up. I feel completely out of control with my life. This nightmare is becoming my reality.

November 1965 ❤

Dear Diary,

I am finally being semi-honest about the double life I'm leading. Both of my families know the truth now. My Danish parents have been incredibly supportive. They're arranging for the adoption. Daddy asked if I wanted to get married but I said no, that this wasn't a good way to start a family. I can sense the fluttering of life inside of me now but I've accepted the fact that I'm not capable of being a mother. "First comes love, then comes marriage, then comes the baby carriage;" those lines make me cry because I didn't do it right. I had such a fantasy in my mind. I'm learning the hard way that life isn't a fairy-tale. My friends haven't said anything about any changes they may have noticed. I've bought one baggy dress and I just pretend I'm my usual happy self. For the December holidays we're traveling to Southern Europe and then they leave in January. I've told them a story about staying longer to become more cultured. What else would I tell them, the truth? I'm too embarrassed and ashamed to admit to anyone that I'm a failure and a fraud. It is almost 1966 and I am terrified.

March 1966 ♥

Dear Diary,

The view from the hospital window is bleak with
skeletal trees standing at attention over the brown
lawn mottled by patches of dirty snow. It has
been an ordeal. I never dreamed I could be this
strong and survive but I had no choice. Once the
other students left for home I started lying about
being married. I wore my opal ring upside down,
like a wedding band, and pretended. At least I
could stop concealing my growing middle and
I even attended a childbirth preparation class.
There was temporary comfort being surrounded by others glowing with their pregancy pride.
I've discovered how dumb I am about my body,
I've never learned anything about sex, much less
pregnancy and birth. I got very sick with toxemia.
I'd only seen the doctor a few times and at my last
appointment I was told to take a taxi with a note
for admission to this big hospital. I was alone,
abandoned once again; ignorant and in a stupor of
denial. High blood pressure meant the baby was
going to be induced and until they stuck a tube in
my arm, I didn't even understand my own reality.
It was when they said the baby was going to be
ok that I sensed any danger. The intense pain of

labor was diminished only during a nightmare I had when they put a mask over my mouth. I saw pink elephants floating around me, telling me I'd been living in a dream and that I was not pregnant. I was told to push but couldn't comprehend and then I was aware of a cry and was told the baby was a girl. I remember being momentarily elated because I knew that her parents already had a son. They could now be a complete family, that fantasy I'd always held for myself. I was now totally alone and missed the baby who had listened to my problems, heart beating within my womb. I never saw her. The sting of my tears were matched by the sorrow in my heart. I've made a vow to myself that whatever it will take, somehow I want to help prevent a repeat of my trauma. This started with a secret. No one else should have to feel this ashamed, sad and alone because of being pregnant and having a baby. In spite of the overly warm hospital room air, I feel a chill and I shudder. I can see beyond the wide wall surrounding the gardens and know now that I have an obligation towards others in the future.

August 1966 🖤

Dear Diary,

We are getting married after all! The electricity
we felt last summer when we first met was there
again as soon as I returned from Denmark. We'd
written a few times during my pregnancy and he
tried to be supportive in his own way. I've told
him a little about my ordeal but I'm not certain
he really understands. I've decided to only think
of the future. Now we're ready to live by "the
rules." I want to graduate from college like I'd
always planned so I'm enrolled in summer school.
I never talk about the baby. I had had this fantasy
about coming home. I would speak frankly and
openly with my family about our baby. What a
silly idea. After all the lying about why I stayed
longer in Denmark, it is not the time for honesty.
The thought of telling the truth has been replaced
by the silence and secret keeping. I do have
dreams about her and wonder if she is ok. It is as
if I left a piece of my soul somewhere, floating in
space. Sometimes I wonder if I'll ever be a mother.
How sad that makes me feel.

September 1967

....

Dear Diary,

What a whirlwind of make believe we've danced
through these past months. Graduation, the
wedding, the honeymoon were nearly picture-card
perfect, but marriage is an altogether different type
of image. I'm reminded of our decision not to be
parents whenever we argue. Learning to make a
marriage work is so hard, I cannot imagine how we
could have been parents too. Somewhere, far away,
she is in good hands growing up within a stable
family, yet I feel a piercing stab of longing and
regret. I secretly saved a copy of the passport photo
that was taken of my baby. It is my only link with
her. I wonder what she looks like now?

June 1970 🖤

Dear Diary,

I've been on an emotional roller-coaster. Daddy died on Father's Day. He didn't get to his only son-in-law's graduation but he did know we'd bought our first home and would be moving away. I weep. He'll never know my children. We never spoke about my decision to keep his grand-daughter from him. We didn't share our feelings whatsoever. Secrets about his mental illness and erratic behavior were kept to protect me. Mom always told me he loved me but I never heard it from his lips and never will. The movers arrive tomorrow to pack our meager belongings from married student housing. We've decided we're ready to become parents. A husband, employment, a home, I wonder if I really am prepared?

January 1971 ♥

Dear Diary,

Getting pregnant isn't easy this time. How ironic!
What if I never do? Have I given away my first
born only to discover I can't have more children? I'm silently in fear since I have no one with
whom I can confide my inner thoughts. I have
made friends with a group of women in town.
We belong to American Association of University
Women (AAUW). Mom is so active with AAUW
and I've always pictured myself joining the
organization once I had my college degree. There
are discussion topics and I've joined one called
"Woman Searching for Self." I certainly feel like
I'm wandering around searching for something
to give meaning to my life. I figured it would be
motherhood. Now I'm beginning to question
that expectation.

August 1971 ❤

Dear Diary,

I can finally shout with pride, I'm pregnant! This is an incredible contrast after getting pregnant too easily the first time, being afraid, ashamed and terrified. I was embarrassed to "confess" to my doctor that I'd already had a baby but he made no judgements. This time we're ready and so excited. I'll let my belly swell, and boast about our impending change of status. This is what I've sacrificed and prayed for, I'll be a mother at last. My joy seems to have no bounds and self-doubts have vanished. My circle of friends through AAUW are all mothers too and I feel like I'm entering a special status as a woman being pregnant. I can talk about my changes with others who have already achieved this rank. I love being pregnant!

March 1972 ❤

Dear Diary,

It's a boy! My dream has come true, I'm finally
a mother. His birth was also induced but having
my husband there was a stark contrast to feeling
deserted by him in 1966. Yet something unexpected has happened to me. How ironic it seems
that after leaving my first born, and denying the
truth about a previous pregnancy, I feel inept and
inadequate. I'd had an expectation that maternal instinct would wash over me and guide me
through each day. It started when we came home
from the security and support of the hospital.
I put my baby in his cozy bed, stood beside
him and thought, now what do I do? From the
triumph and exhilaration of birth, I've plunged
to being overwhelmed and exhausted. I am alone
and frightened. The truth is I'm clueless about
this new job and as a couple we're nearly hopeless.
At our baby's first two-week check-up, we discovered that he had not gained any weight and he
had an inguinal hernia. Surgery was mentioned,
supplemental bottles were added to my obviously
insufficient nursing routine, and we walked out
of the doctor's office in a daze. I began to notice
a pain in my stomach. Who has ever heard of a

baby causing an ulcer? From then on, the tension has mounted. My husband knows less than I do and keeps expecting to learn from me. At one point he stood in the doorway as I tried to nurse and said I was starving his child. I cried and he turned away in frustration. The baby's schedule is like a Ferris wheel in high gear, whirling and spinning. I feel like a damp washcloth being wrung out for the hundredth time as I nurse constantly. When I attended a nursing mother's group and confessed that I've been using supplemental bottles, I could feel their glares of disapproval not to mention their silence of disgust. Mom came down for a few days but couldn't or didn't want to stay. I'm so incredibly alone. What am I going to do to survive this hideous existence?

May 1972 ♥

Dear Diary,

I'm so blue in-between the surges of love for my newborn. I'm crying over stupid things like getting black stains on the sheets when doing the wash. I stood in front of the washing machine holding the villainous socks amidst a pile of dirty laundry with tears pouring down my face. I feel paralyzed by guilt that I should be able to cope and function like all those other moms. Isn't this why I delayed being a mother so I could do it right this time? At 10 weeks, the pediatrician told me to start the baby on solids because he still isn't gaining weight. I truly am a failure as a nursing mom. He seems content, but I'm not okay. The other day I fainted from trying to contain a pain in my chest. The doctor checked me for physical ailments then sent me home. He never asked how I was feeling emotionally so I certainly didn't volunteer my sense of inadequacy, mood swings, poor sleeping, lack of concentration, and anxiousness. Maybe things will get better with time.

August 1972 ♥

Dear Diary,

Guess what, I'm still alive and so is our son. It seems like a miracle but my life as a mother has improved. I've made friends with other new mothers at a child study group through AAUW who have helped me realize I'm not crazy or alone. It is a form of therapy, I guess. We've been using our intellect and frequent gatherings to share mutual concerns and sometimes we laugh out-loud. My stomach and headaches are not as frequent probably because I'm sleeping and eating better now. I still can't get over how easy I thought this was going to be. My friends agree that reading all those expert opinions on how to parent isn't nearly as helpful as our sitting in the park sharing our experiences. Once I let my mask of smiles slip and I was partially honest about myself, it made such a difference in my behavior and mood. That inner shame I feel about my secret past won't allow me to ever tell the whole true.

March 1973 🖤

Dear Diary,

It is his first birthday! What an amazing year we've
shared as a family. I've kept a "first moments"
list of his physical developments; teeth, crawling,
sleeping, eating, walking, talking. To be a witness
to these miracles is worth the sleepless nights and
torments of self-doubt. He is clearly a loving indi-
vidual, energetic and bright. I'm in awe that my lack
of maternal instinct and self-confidence in those
beginning weeks did not damage him. He is loved
and treasured and it is reciprocated. My reflections
include fear, dread, near panic and pending loss
tangled into a web of patience, pride and stubborn
determination. That murky soup of emotional con-
trasts must be rather typical for motherhood. We've
received birthday cards and messages from family
and friends. My niece wrote to her new cousin
"You're growing up in a very strange world of today
and tomorrows. It has a lot of good sides and a
few bad ones too. You won't always escape the bad
things, nor can those who love you try to shield you
forever. Life is full of puzzles, many of which you
may never understand."

January 1974 ♥

Dear Diary,

We're trying to get pregnant again. I want our son to have a sibling and I want to raise more children. Am I crazy? Being a mother is so demanding and draining and yet, there is this piece of me needing another baby. I survived those darker moments during his early months and now I can only really remember the happy times. Our son is so active, I swear he could generate electricity if we could put him on a treadmill and harness his energy. I think I'm prepared for the unexpected next time around. Now I just hope I can be blessed with another chance to be a mommy.

Dear Diary,

I'm eight months pregnant and so excited. We went to Disneyland as a last hurrah before the baby comes. While riding the steamboat my son gave me a big hug around my huge belly and said, "mom, I hope the baby grows up to be just like me!" What a loving, self-confident little man he is. I secretly worry about my ability to share the love I feel for him with his unborn sibling. I wonder if other mothers feel like this? Is there a boundary around a mother's love? Actually, I'm more frightened by the memory of lost sleep. For good luck I stroke my bulging abdomen in circles and say aloud "you will sleep through the night" over and over. It can't hurt and maybe he/she is listening. Sleep deprivation is painful. I think I can handle any stress if I'm allowed to sleep. We'll find out!

February 1975 ♥

Dear Diary,

A girl! My tears of joy at the sight of my beautiful daughter are mixed up the sting of memories of her lost sister. I've been blessed to have been given this second chance to raise a girl. My feelings of elation were dashed the day we were taking her home by the doctor's announcement of her jaundice. Yet, the homecoming was perfect since big brother and grandma were there to welcome her with kisses and hugs. But her condition only got worse and those pains in my stomach and heart I'd had 3 and 9 years before are back. She nurses so well, we call her "super sucker" but I lie awake wondering if she's going to die. My moods come and go. After all, maybe I'm being punished for my previous sin. I can't talk to anyone about my fears of losing her but if we do, it will be all my fault.

My secret keeps haunting me.

March 1975 🖤

Dear Diary,

My baby girl is out of danger! Her jaundice has
abated after weeks of pricking her tiny pink
heels for blood tests. I'm not obsessing about her
now and will try to stay happy. Her big brother
continues to challenge and exhaust me but we're
bonded so tightly it feels like silly putty in a cup.
He can pull and stretch me in all directions and
then I bounce back into a blob. I hope to keep
from reaching a melt down point and flowing out
of control with my emotions. We enrolled him in
a pre-school after the baby was born against the
advice of others saying he needs to be at home so
he doesn't feel displaced by the baby. He seemed
ready so off he went to "big-boy school." I felt
guilty so I decided to volunteer one morning
and told him I'd be there. He responded, "no,
mommy, it is my school." I ignored him. It isn't
easy getting everyone ready but after first taking
him to school, nursing the baby and leaving her
at a girl friends I went back to volunteer. At first
he didn't notice me as I helped sort papers in a

corner across the brightly decorated playroom. I felt fulfilled as a "perfect" mom until he looked up, saw me and shouted "get out of my school." This piece of silly putty blushed and retreated. I cried as I drove myself back to get the baby, I don't exactly know why. Maternal attachments and their accompanying emotions are incredibly complex. My girl friends' support continues to be a source of comfort. I am reminded by their similar stories that I'm not alone.

July 1977

Dear Diary,

My vow of long ago has taken on a form and
direction. I have a purpose now beyond being a
mother and a wife and my energy has come from
that unspoken force in the back of my mind. I
still haven't told my friends that I gave away our
first baby because I feel such shame and embar-
rassment surrounding my unresolved guilt. My
friends and I have launched a community-based,
grassroots, self-help parent support program. We
were funded by a grant from AAUW. It is an idea
born from our own experiences and needs. We
have named it Postpartum Education for Parents,
PEP for short, and laughed about not calling the
organization "afterbirth." The word postpartum
is not in the public's vocabulary yet but it is that
period of time from birth through the first year
of a baby's life. We have become social pioneers
by starting a Warm Line. The idea originated
from our confessions that there had been times
after becoming first time mothers that we might
have called the "hot line" in town but we never
had the nerve to do that. There is such a stigma
to the thought that we were in any type of crisis.
What we had felt were "normal crazy" thoughts.

We each had wished for someone to call, share worries and discuss options without being judged. So that is what we've designed. This vision is a partial fulfillment of my vow. The next step is to start groups so new parents can get together and share in person. I was the volunteer on duty when the first phone call came through the answering service. All I did was reassure the caller that what she was feeling and describing was okay. When she asked me how old my children were her response to my answer was "oh, you've made it, I guess I will too." It is so simple just being there for someone. Privately I moan to myself, why, oh why hadn't there been anyone for me after giving birth. It isn't normal for women to feel so alone.

April 1979 ❤

Dear Diary,

One of my personal goals (a piece of my vow) has been to educate society about the role that volunteers and self help plays in the prevention of problems. So, guess what?! I had my article about starting PEP published! It is so exciting to see my name and our story in print. The title the magazine, *American Baby*, gave my story is "Parents Helping Parents." We've been getting publicity about PEP in a few newspapers and magazines so my friends and I wrote a book about how we got started. We've called it *A Guide for Establishing a Parent Support Program in Your Community.* It is becoming clear that I've found my "niche."

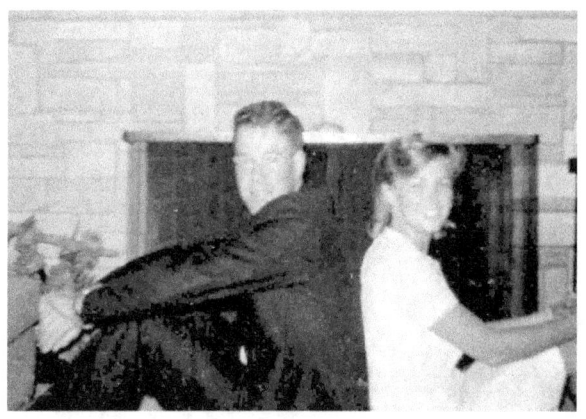

Summer love, August 1965

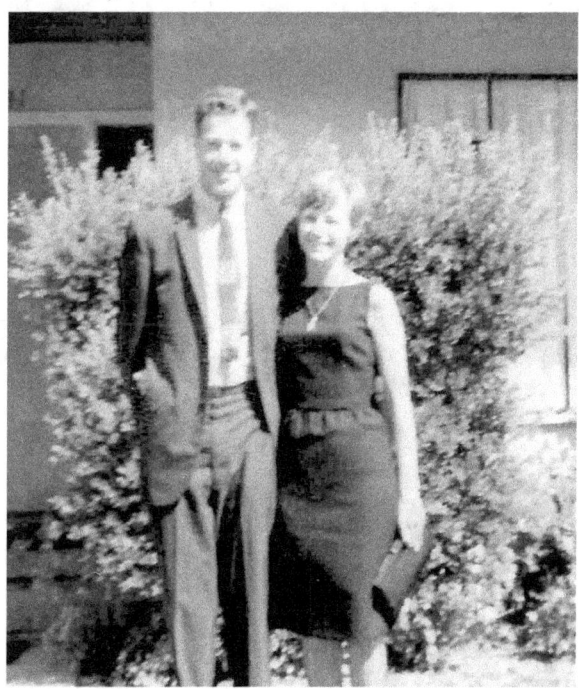

Engagement photo, August 1966

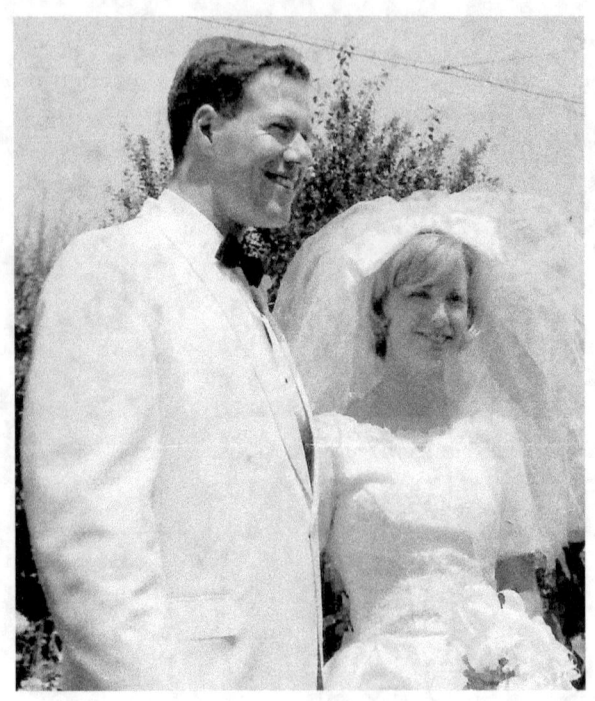

It is official, September 1967

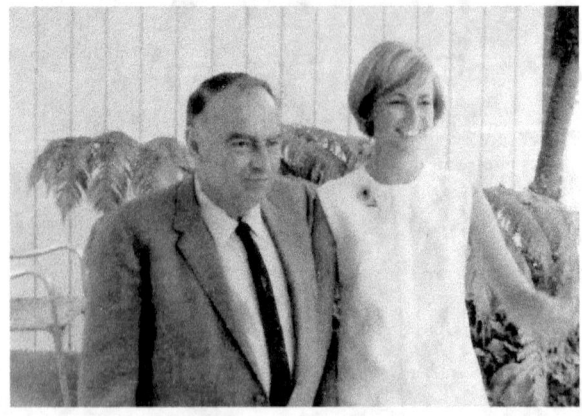

Daddy and me, June 1970

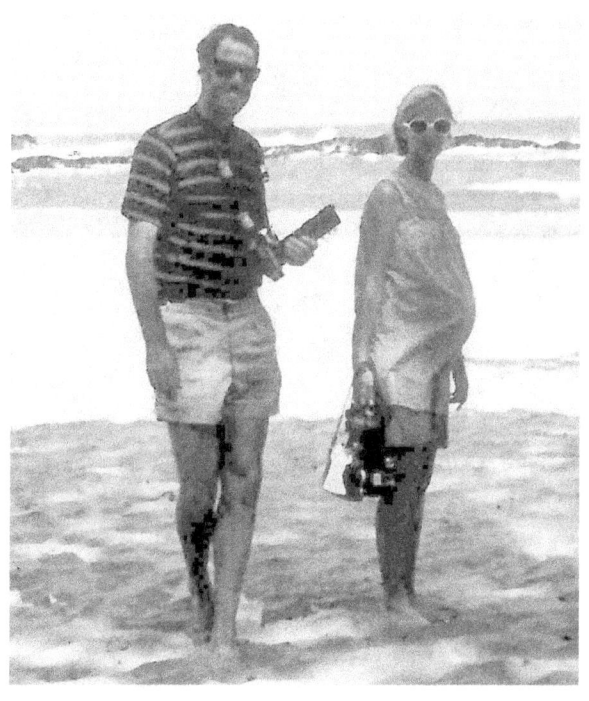

Barefoot and pregnant, 1972

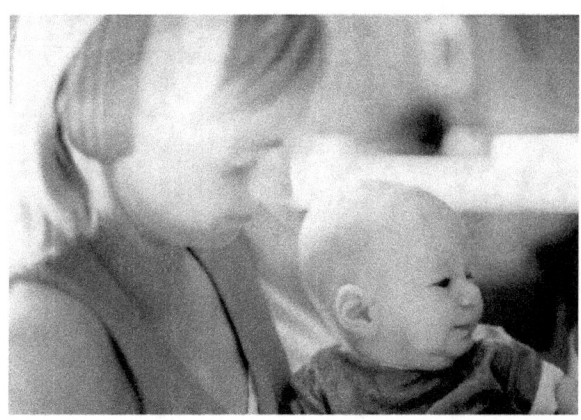

Mother and son, 1972

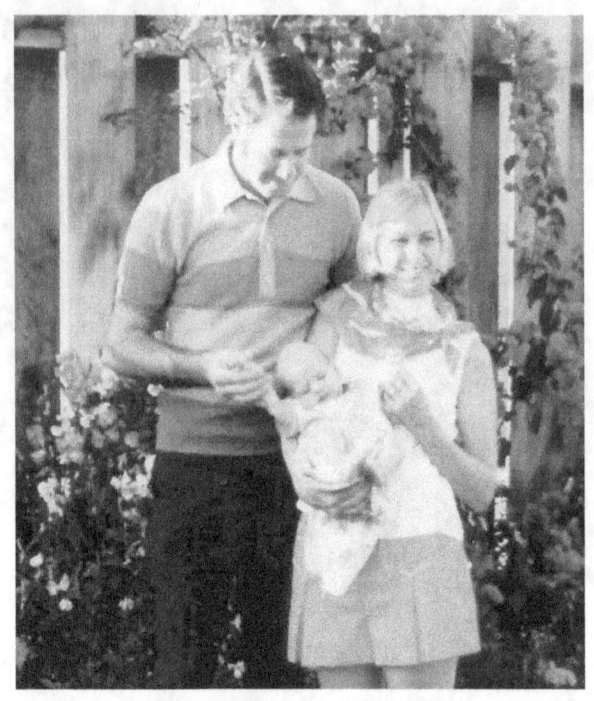

Clueless parents, May 1972

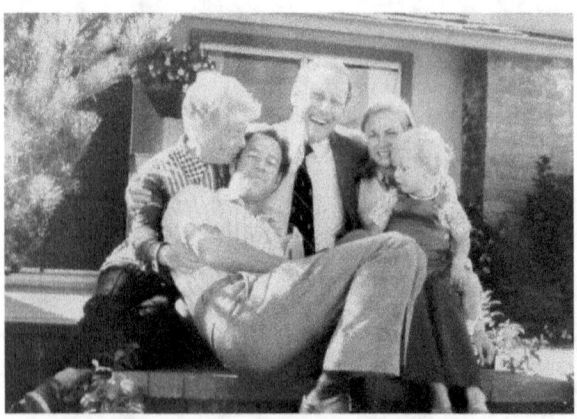

Happy clan, January 1974

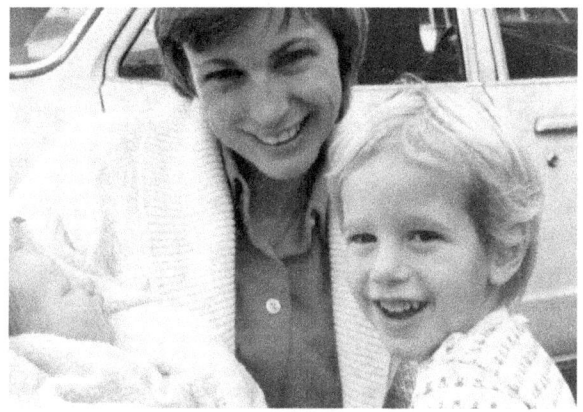

Little sister, February 1975

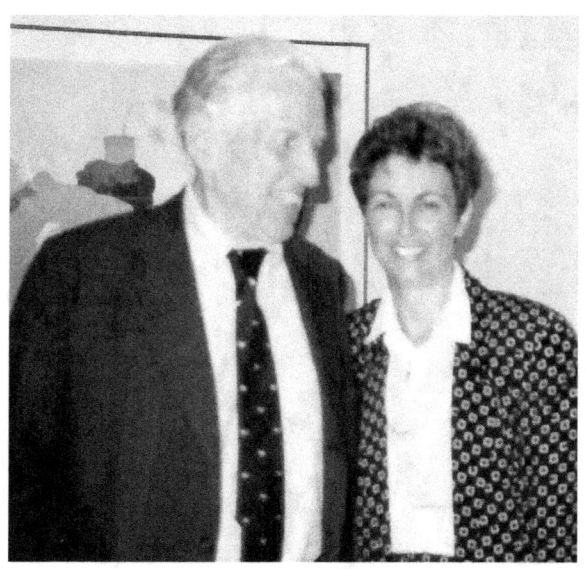

With Dr. Hamilton

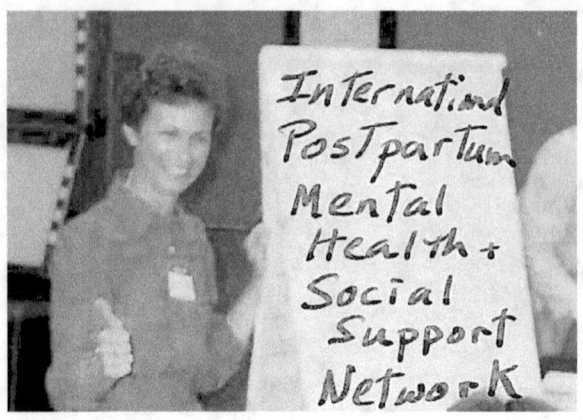

Birth of a movement, June 1987

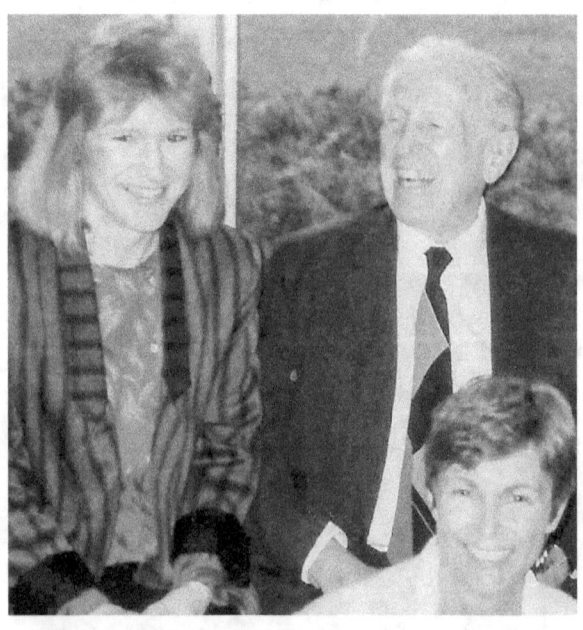

With Carol Dix and James Hamilton, July 1988

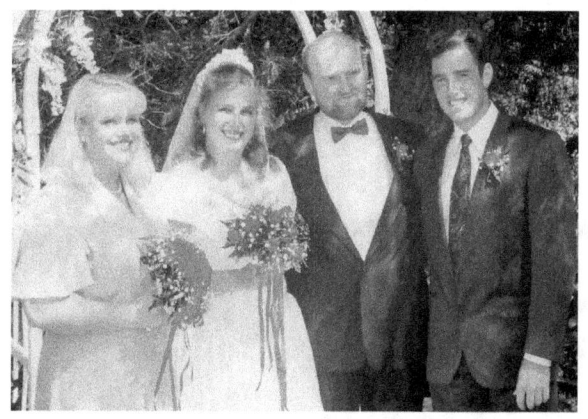

Complete family, January 1994

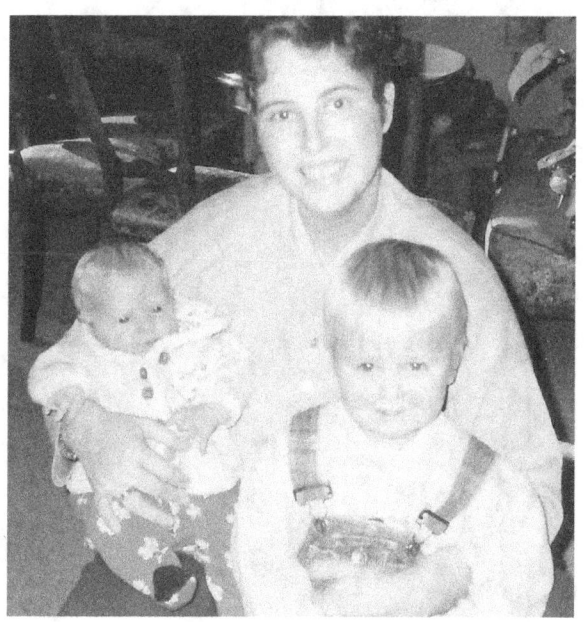

Gift of the next generation, October 1999

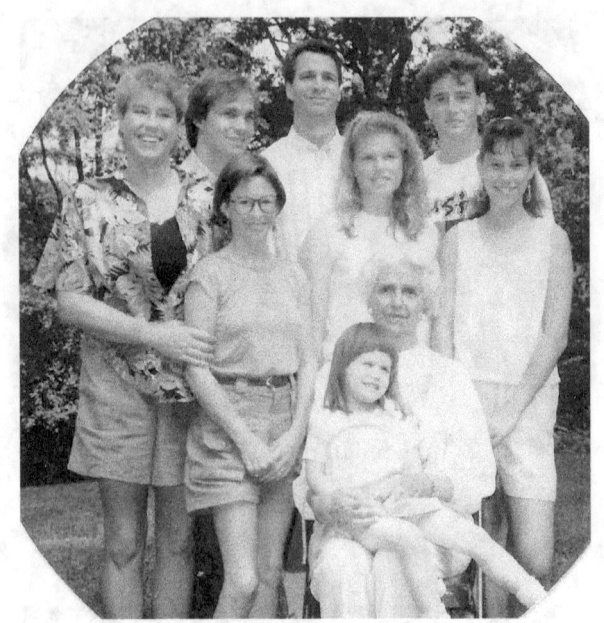

My mother and her grandchildren, 1990

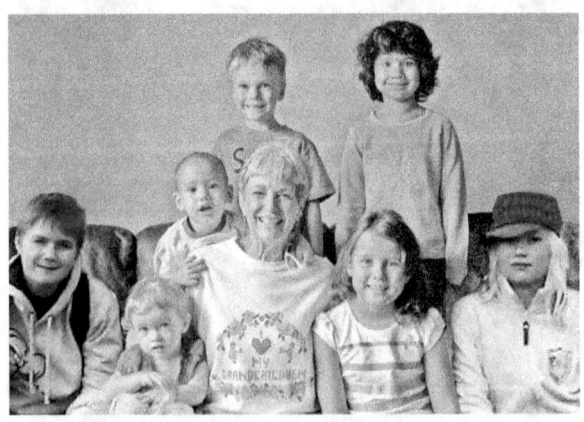

With my grandchildren, 2010

March 1980 ♥

Dear Diary,

You'll never believe this, but I was featured in
a national magazine called *Parents* in an article
called "Six Women Who Can Help You Cope."
It is all about PEP and I feel so proud but a little
embarrassed too. After all, I did not start PEP
alone. The main point is to get the word out and
it seems to be happening. I've also applied for a
personal grant from AAUW to conduct a research
study about other postpartum support groups.
I've become a member of the local Junior League
too. Another project I've helped launch is about
childcare. What an amazing era it is for me as
a young woman and mother. I see my gender
continuing the struggle our foremothers started
in the previous century. My mother gave me a tee
shirt with the slogan "it's great to be a woman"
on the back. She is my role model and I want her
to be proud of me.

July 1981 ♥

Dear Diary,

I'm using my brain again! I've been so busy this past year working on a project called "A Study of the Dynamics and Development of Postpartum Support Groups." Last April I was notified that I'd been awarded that grant from AAUW. I was inspired to try for the grant after receiving over 400 letters requesting information after my article was published in 1979. My intent was to determine if there should be a national network of similar postpartum support groups. I heard back from 68 of the 120 groups I contacted and then I compared their histories and services and financial backing. There seems to be a growing interest in providing services and resources to families, however, only a few work specifically with maternal mental health. Now that it is completed, I wonder what will come of my study.

July 1982 🖤

Dear Diary,

I've linked with a new national organization
called the Family Resource Coalition based in
Chicago. They are doing what I envisioned in
my AAUW study by starting a national clearing-
house of community based, parent support organizations. Their leader, Bernice Weissbourd,
is my mentor. I want to see a postpartum parent
support group in every community just as we
have in Santa Barbara. The Coalition's newsletter
is printing an article I wrote about PEP and I'll
attend the first national conference on family
support. This is progress.

January 1984 ♥

Dear Diary,

It is amazing how one phone call can open doors
and bring unimagined opportunity. Carol Dix
is an author. She is living in New York City now
and writing a book on postpartum depression.
She wants my help in distributing a questionnaire
to new parents and found PEP in her search for
contacts. Our conversation made me realize how
little I really understand about depression especially when she asked specifically if I'd ever heard
of a Dr. James Hamilton or something called the
Marcé Society. Her answer to my negative reply
was "well, if you haven't then no one has." She
gave me Dr. Hamilton's telephone number in San
Francisco and I decided to call, introduce myself
and tell him about PEP. His response was warm
and welcoming. He asked me to send information
about PEP to him. Sometimes I can't believe I
have the nerve to take such risks but then I get
this surge of courage from remembering my vow.

March 1984 ♥

Dear Diary,

I received a personal letter from Dr. Hamilton
and a copy of his book he wrote in 1962 called
Postpartum Psychiatric Problems. It a thrill and
honor that he is interested in our program.

He has invited me to an August Marcé meeting to
speak about a "normal sample" of mothers. I am
especially puzzled by what he means by saying,
"This may be one long continuum. You may
already have information on the effect of suppres-
sion of lactation, done by people who don't want
to nurse, but who are not intentionally avoiding
postpartum distress." It is abundantly clear that
I have a great deal to learn about how psychiatry
fits into obstetrics and parenting.

August 1984 ♥

Dear Diary,

I've just returned from meeting the most remarkable professionals from around the world. I'm overwhelmed by the complexity of the information I heard. I'm beginning to wonder if what I've felt off and on during my childbearing years is more than psychological. It feels scary to think that I might have had a real illness.Dr. Hamilton had faith in me so I gulped back my insecurity and spoke out. My talk was called A System for Action and I had only 5 minutes to describe PEP and the role of non-medical, self-help support volunteers. I sold several of our PEP books, one to a psychiatrist in Australia. It is looking like my original idea of starting a national network has become international. I feel that my dream of helping other people avoid what I've gone through is starting to become a reality.

April 1985 🖤

Dear Diary,

I'm turning 40 this year, a time of transitions. An opportunity came my way to take on a part time paid position as the Director of the Santa Barbara Birth Resource Center (BRC). I'm a "new me." I'd been asked to think of someone who might want to apply for the position and I thought to myself, why not me? It will be a challenge and I'm eager to watch myself tackle parenting issues from a new perspective. I've been trying to create change as a volunteer, maybe being in an employed position will afford new opportunities. We'll see, wish me good luck!

January 1986 ❤

Dear Diary,

I love being in charge! Carol Dix author of
The New Mother Syndrome came and gave a
lecture as a fundraiser for the BRC. It was an
honor to stand before a large audience in the
hospital's auditorium and introduce her as my
friend. She is the one who has opened my eyes to
postpartum depression. I'm also working closely
with a few PEP volunteers on a research project.
We've designed a telephone and written survey of
the professionals in the community to develop a
referral list. Nancy Lee has become a particularly
dedicated friend. She is motivated by knowing
a woman who suffered from severe postpartum
depression. We've started writing a brochure
after realizing the only ones available are from
England. I'm witnessing progress in my own
search for the truth. It still feels like a puzzle
but I have no doubt that I'm on track towards
solving it.

Dear Diary,

This is the speech I'm going to give as a member of a panel of local experts on Postpartum Adjustment.

"I am here tonight as a mother and a resource person. I have been involved with this subject intimately for nearly 15 years. It is hard to believe that number because it seems like only yesterday that we brought our son home from the "perfect" delivery. You can guess correctly that our world changed forever the day the hospital honeymoon was over and we faced our postpartum adjustment. I won't go into my story or the others that led to the forming of PEP ten years ago. I am not a medical expert, a social worker or counselor but I am the voice of those women and their partners who are silent. I am able to articulate the realities of what becoming a parent is all about. It is, in fact, a mixed blessing. I feel strongly that everyone experiences some form of negative reaction which balances the joys of birth and childrearing. No one is immune to postpartum adjustment. Each of us will react in his or her own way and in his or her own time to the challenges of parenthood. What I've said so far is not controversial or radical so why am I saying this? Because #1, very few people have been honest enough to confront the myths of parenthood that our society perpetuates. #2, hardly anyone is talking about the mental health half of our bodies. And #3, because for hundreds of years medical science has been baffled by and unable to adequately explain exactly why and how it is that some women, 1 in 10, experience such a negative reaction to childbirth that they require professional care. Tonight you are witnessing a profound historical event. I am proud to announce the publication of the first American brochure of its kind called "The Emotional You." It was written by Nancy Lee and myself and printed by a grant from the March of Dimes. It will be sold nation wide to combat the myths surrounding motherhood. You are participating in the birth of a new age of understanding of women's mental health. I am determined to change the past and forge a new future that includes the emotional half of ourselves. I believe that the stability of families rests on this issue. I believe that we, as consumers, must speak up and ask that professionals listen to our feelings. We will no longer be silent, but vigilant in our need to care for ourselves, our partners and our children.

I pledge to no longer cry in silence and wipe my tears pretending that I am not overwhelmed, lonely or frightened. I can relate to each one of you whatever your state of mental health. Together we will ask questions, seek help if needed, and work towards a better tomorrow." I wonder what the response will be to those lofty words...

June 1987 🖤

Dear Diary,

After three years of traveling in England for meetings and learning from the scientists I decided it was time to bring together those of us who have been working with the mothers and their families as self-help supporters. Dr. Hamilton has agreed to speak at the First Annual Postpartum Mental Health Conference in Santa Barbara. Two Canadian postpartum groups are sending presenters so it is truly an international affair. My goal is to lead the formation of a network of social support groups. Twenty-one years ago I made a vow to do "something." While I am still uncertain of the fate of my first offspring, I am certain that I will not abandon this creation.

July 1988

Dear Diary,

I'm back from our second annual meeting on women's mental health. It was held in Princeton, New Jersey. I'll be writing the bylaws for becoming an incorporated not for profit organization called Postpartum Support International. Dr. Hamilton suggested that name and it will be called PSI for short. I've also started leading a postpartum depression support group in town. The more I listen to other women the more I learn. I'm beginning to realize I have yet to deal with my own denial about my first baby. It is too painful and embarrassing to talk about it but I'm being asked by more and more women "what happened to you?"

August 1989 ♥

Dear Diary,

It has been a hectic summer but exhilarating as
I traveled to Kansas City, Chicago and Seattle
giving talks on postpartum depression. Two
important emotional turning points happened at
my last stop. I invited my niece to stay with me
during the annual PSI conference. I decided it
was time to tell someone in my family the truth
about my year in Denmark. She is only five years
younger than I am so we've been raised almost
like sisters. It was a relief to share my secret after
all these years of silence. Her reaction was loving
and supportive. I was elected President of PSI at
this meeting and that is another positive step in
my personal growth.

October 1991 🖤

Dear Diary,

I celebrated my 46th birthday with my Danish
"parents" this year and have asked their assistance
in helping me find my first born. I can't believe that
I finally have taken this enormous leap. They are
most enthusiastic about my request. My husband
knows about this decision but not the children.
I told them each when they turned 13 years old
about my first baby and their initial reaction was
anger and then acceptance. I'll wait and see what
develops before I tell anyone else. It is absolutely
terrifying to contemplate what I've begun. I fear
there might be bad news but I have to find out the
truth. I've lived too long with this burden, I can't
stand the weight of the pain any longer.

July 1992 ♥

Dear Diary,

It happened, at last. I finally know that she is
alive, very well and happy. I've returned from
a conference in Sweden. On my way there I
stayed over in Copenhagen and learned about my
Danish baby girl. She agreed to receive a letter
from me and so I wrote one asking her to forgive
me. I hold in my hand her response. "Dear Jane,
thank you for your letter, it wasn't such a shock
as you thought. My father asked me a while ago
if it was OK for you to contact me, so I was more
or less prepared. I have always known that I was
adopted and that my mother was from USA. I'm
happy to know that your life turned out all right,
that you married Terry and got two beautiful
kids. I can only agree with you, concerning your
decision 26 years ago. You did what was right
and best for me. I have the most loving parents

and have had a beautiful childhood. Tragically I lost my mother 1 ½ years ago, but I still got my father and we are very close. I'm curious to know about my roots, so I hope for us to correspond and perhaps to meet in the future." I have found a profound sense of peace. I didn't realize how troubled I've been all these years until this heaviness vanished from my soul. The truth has set me free. I can only hope that I haven't hurt anyone else I love from my actions.

July 1993 ♥

Dear Diary,

We've met and it is a miracle to witness and watch as we adjust to the dynamics of this adventure. We're each experiencing our own emotional reactions as we explore this new relationship. I'm amazed and amused by our similarities. We find the same jokes funny and have dislikes in common. There is a powerful biological connection. She calls me Jane and we've talked about her deep love for her parents. Even if we never meet again I'm relieved she knows about her biological background. She has answers to questions which she'd asked but no one else could answer. That feels good.

July 1994 ❤

Dear Diary,

A wedding! Yes, we now have a Danish son-in-law and have hosted our first family marriage ceremony and celebration. Whoever could have guessed that I'd see my younger children standing beside the baby I never held at her wedding. It was a highly charged emotional moment and I let my tears flow. What joy!

June 1995 🖤

Dear Diary,

I "went" back to school to get a Masters degree in Psychology. For the past 4 years I've been doing independent study through California Coast University. I never left my house because it is a "long distance learning" program. This was perfect for me since I've been able to run PSI from our home on a daily basis and study at the same time. I'm especially proud of the thesis I wrote called "The Mental Heath Assessment Practices of Health Care Providers for Pregnant and Postpartum Parents." My objectives were:

1) To identify the current level of knowledge, attitudes, and actual assessment practices about maternal mental health of the pre and post natal health care practitioners.

2) To compare the results of this 1994 study with the findings in 1991 to determine a trend in professionals' practices.

The Study Design examined the routine practices of 58 physicians and nurses, their education, and their opinions about their knowledge about prenatal and postpartum mood and anxiety disorders.

An updated screening checklist questionnaire designed and used in Sacramento County, California in 1991 was used in this replication of that survey for Santa Barbara and Ventura Counties, California in 1994.

My results showed that the majority of the health care practitioners were educated in their medical and/or nursing schools, and/or through post-graduate seminars and that they did discuss the predictive factors of maternal mental illness with their patients. Their median number of years in practice was 13.1. Slightly more than one half of the primary care providers were satisfied that they have sufficient knowledge about postpartum mental health. The results revealed that the professionals did not use a screening tool to evaluate their patients for depression, anxiety and stress. Only two obstetricians, three nurse practitioners, and three postpartum nurses responded that they use a particular postpartum questionnaire. All of the mental health issues were discussed more often after delivery than during pregnancy. A high percentage of the respondents did inquire into the social support system of the woman, did involve her partner in a treatment plan, and did refer their patients to mental health professionals and support groups. These professionals were discussing the mild emotional reactions to pregnancy and birth, but they did not uniformly inform their patients, through literature or discussion, about the major postpartum mood and anxiety disorders. A high percentage of the practitioners discussed the blues and depression but few discussed panic disorder and psychosis. An equally high percentage (96.2%) inquired about the woman's previous history of mental illness as those who discussed the blues. Nearly as many asked about her family's psychiatric history. Only slightly more than half asked about a history of premenstrual syndrome. More than three quarters inquired about support for the woman during pregnancy and postpartum.

My conclusions: Health care providers are actively concerned, to some degree, with the mental health of their pregnant and postpartum patients but they do not, however, routinely discuss the major maternal mental health disorders either during pregnancy or after delivery. There is a need for an effort to encourage health care practitioners to use a standardized, written screening tool during pregnancy and postpartum.

October 1999

Dear Diary,

I am a grandmother now. I have held my grand-
babies and reached the status of matriarch. My
mother died in March 1998 and I grieved for our
families' loss. She was my mentor and best friend.
We were extremely close and yet I could never talk
to her about my first pregnancy and its repercus-
sions on my life. It took me twenty-five years to
realize I had to take care of myself, by myself,
even though I feared hurting my mother. I did
hurt her by reawakening that shame in my past but
in the end she was able to acknowledge another
granddaughter and her fourth great grandson. I've
learned through the years that there are two major
barriers to finding a life of peace. They are denial
and ignorance. We can tackle most of life's obsta-
cles if we seek knowledge yet that is not sufficient.
I'd become educated about depression but it took
confronting the truth in my past before I could
conquer my hidden sadness. I had a secret but the
truth has helped me heal. It has been a painful
journey but I am a wiser woman because of this
path. I like myself and my life now. Thanks, Diary
for listening. I don't need you any longer.

Epilogue

During the past fifteen years, life has been less intense. I welcomed in the twenty first century with my family while on holiday in Guatemala. No one worried about computers crashing as we climbed ruins in the jungle of an ancient civilization.

Our son was married in 2000, and our younger daughter in 2003. Three granddaughters and two grandsons were born. I'm pleased to say that none of the new parents suffered from pregnancy or postpartum distress or depression. The mothers were mothered by their devoted husbands, surrounded by extended family, support networks, and friends. They had everything we lacked. I had to adapt to a new role and learn to keep my mouth shut. Happily, the psychological dimension of grandparenthood included the emotional high without the physicality of sleep deprivation. I will confess though that sometimes I did cry as I struggled to find balance in the changing hierarchy of the family.

After seventeen years, Postpartum Support International's office moved out of our home. It was a tense transition that required trial, error, countless hours of training, and staff interventions. I saw myself floundering as a founder. I was no longer in charge but not certain of my new role. We got a new home telephone number. It was a relief not receiving calls of crisis and distress day in and day out. My "baby" had left the nest. Now what? PSI had been my career; yet I wasn't really ready to retire from the world I'd conceived, delivered and nurtured.

Outside of Santa Barbara, I maintained my membership with the Marcé Society, and of course, PSI. I continued to travel the world and participated in conferences on maternal mental health. Locally, I joined new organizations, and made new acquaintances. I now had more time to take music lessons, work in our garden, and best of all, be available to help our children with the grandchildren. I tried to follow my own "steps to wellness."

The truth is that I continue to struggle with mild depression. The one tell-tale sign I have when I'm "sinking" is feeling as though I don't have any friends. Of course, I have plenty of friends, and I know I'm not alone. My mind says one thing but my brain chemistry takes me to a sad place. Thankfully, I've gained insight and recognize when I need to ask for help.

As I've aged and become wiser, I can acknowledge the truth about myself. I am who I am, and appreciate my journey through six decades. Facing my seventies, and who knows how many more years ahead, I feel blessed as I greet each day, and acknowledge those who have guided, and accompanied me. With the positive feedback I've received about my work, I realize my example of pain has inspired others to reach beyond hurt, and contribute to a purpose greater than oneself.